Resistance Band Exercises

24 Stretching and Strength Training Workouts You
Can Do at Home or On the Go to Build Muscle,
Lose Weight and Improve Body Fitness

By

Teri Wheeler

Disclaimer

This book offers knowledgeable and trustworthy information on the subject area discussed. Nevertheless, the opinions presented in this work belong solely to the author and are not intended to be considered expert advice or counsel. The reader is therefore accountable for his/ her own decision.

Contents

Introduction

Resistance bands are large, flexible, and stretchy bands for maintaining physical body fitness with a huge versatile application, such as for stretching, strength, workouts, mobility, and warm-ups.

All fitness levels can benefit from resistance bands. Resistance bands are excellent for beginners to develop their muscles and strength along with their flexibility and mobility. For intermediate and advanced fitness levels, resistance bands can be utilized in working out efficiently whether you have no access to weights, are traveling, or prefer to work out at home. Moreover, because they are significantly less physically demanding on the body, they make logical sense if you wish to take a break from lifting weights, allowing your joints to have some rest.

Everyone must undergo an exercise to help strengthen their muscles at least three times a week. Undergoing strength and stretching exercises using the resistance band helps in the development of body muscles, thereby helping you perform your regular daily and strenuous activities without burning out. If you're undergoing any strength training or rehab program, such as for leg or knee injuries, then a resistance band is a perfect addition to include in your workout routine. They come in several types, colors, and levels of resistance. Resistance bands are portable, making them ideal for home use, and can be taken with you anywhere you go, which also makes them great for on-the-go exercises.

In this book, I have taken out time to discuss several resistance band exercises covering the full body. legs, glutes, chest, shoulders, arms, and core that you can try at home or on the go to enhance your strength, build your muscles, burn fat and improve your overall body fitness and well-being. The exercises have been designed so that you can easily implement them on your own. Needless to say, you'd be properly acquainted with every detail you need to know to make the most out of the exercises.

So, let's get started right away.

Chapter 1

Fundamentals of Resistance Bands

What are Resistance Bands?

Rubber strips with elastic properties are known as resistance bands, and they are used to give the body some resistance while exercising. You could target individual muscle groups like the quadriceps, hamstrings, chest, shoulders, glutes, biceps, and triceps with resistance bands, or you could perform exercises that work on the entire body. Therefore, resistance bands, like free weights, are capable of targeting any muscle group.

Resistance bands come in single strips and long and short loops (like large elastic bands), each of which has a specific application. Each band offers a range of resistance levels since they are elastic, and as you stretch them, the precise resistance they produce improves. The individual bands can be utilized for a variety of activities because of their adjustable resistance. All skill levels can use them; seasoned gym-goers can choose a tougher level of resistance band, while beginners can use a lighter level of resistance band. Resistance bands offer some of the best value for money in the exercise equipment sector, are lightweight, inexpensive compared to most exercise equipment, and are very portable.

Benefits of Resistance Bands

The good news is that the well-known bands have advantages for everyone, regardless of your physical condition or fitness objectives. In fact, a study published in the Journal of Physical Therapy Science reveals that using resistance bands on a regular basis can enhance balance, mobility, gait function, and fall efficacy in older adults.

Let's now delve deeper into the advantages of resistance bands.

- **Tone and build up**

Resistance bands cause your muscles to contract and become more tense as they stretch. The resistance increases in intensity as the band is stretched, making the exercise harder. Additionally, you can increase the resistance by holding the resistance band in a way that increases the tension by bringing your hands closer together when performing arm movements.

- **Add support rather than just resistance**

Your success with challenging activities can be aided by using resistance bands. For individuals who want to improve their pull-up technique, you can simply attach the resistance band to the bar and place it under your foot or knee to switch up to an unassisted mode. Your weight is supported by the band when you complete the pull-up exercise while using the band, which makes it easier to complete.

- **Really good for stretching**

Ever suffered from neck or back pain? Through certain effective stretching techniques, resistance bands can help relieve upper body pain. Sit on the floor with your legs outstretched and wrap the resistance band around your feet for a terrific upper back stretch. Gently bend your back away from your feet by grabbing the resistance band's sides at shoulder width. When stretching out after working out, you can also utilize resistance bands. Resistance bands will enable you to gradually lengthen your limbs and relieve any muscular strain.

- **Portable and lightweight**

For those looking to work out while traveling, these bands are the ideal accessory. Due to their exceptional lightness, they may be stowed away in either hand luggage or a carry-on.

- **Beneficial for recovering from injuries and good for almost everyone**

Similar to how weights work your muscles, resistance bands put pressure on your body through contractions that stabilize and control the movement you want. But unlike weights, resistance bands don't get their resistance from gravity. In certain exercises, the body can move and increase its range of motion (e.g., lift the arms higher in a sidearm lift).

For those recovering from a sports- or muscle-related injury, resistance bands have been a mainstay. This is so that your joints and everything else are safe since resistance bands don't apply pressure in the same way that weights do. Furthermore, since many stretches and exercises can be performed while seated, resistance bands are an effective workout tool for people of any age and fitness level.

- **Keeps bones and muscles stronger**

Similar to how resistance bands help your muscles, they also help your bones become stronger. In general, strength training can help your bones grow more cells and become denser, which will help to prevent diseases like osteoporosis and back pain. Resistance bands help to jump-start bone-building because they add extra resistance to strength exercises. Exercises performed with resistance bands have a lower impact than those performed without them, which is better for your joints.

- **Affordable**

Resistance bands are reasonably priced, ranging from $5 to $10. Just keep in mind that the exercises will become more difficult as the band becomes thicker and more resistant. To ensure that you always have a selection of different resistances, choose a variety pack.

- **Loss of weight**

The most important aspect of fat loss is energy balance. If you burn more calories through exercise than you consume through food and drink, you will lose weight and fat. Although changing your diet and habits will be the most crucial factor in fat loss, exercise is also extremely important.

Building muscle through resistance training will increase the number of calories your body burns all day long, even when you're at rest. Nutrient partitioning is a concept that explains how exercise will encourage your food to go more toward nourishing and replenishing your muscles rather than being stored as fat.

Exercise also burns calories, which is perhaps the most obvious benefit. Utilizing resistance bands increases the body's resistance, resulting in a greater level of effort and greater calorie and energy expenditure. Resistance bands can undoubtedly help you lose weight, provided your diet is balanced.

Who Can Use Resistance Bands?

After reading about the advantages of resistance bands, it should be obvious that everyone can utilize them to achieve their fitness objectives. Here are some specific groups who ought to use them and why.

- **Anyone Seeking To Improve Muscle**

In order to provide your muscles with a novel and complex stimulus for growth, you can utilize resistance bands in place of dumbbells and machines if you're trying to increase your muscular size and strength.

Additionally, you can include them in barbell exercises to up the difficulty and neuromuscular performance.

- **Everyone Who Wishes To Lose Weight**

When you combine a good diet, exercise, and strength training, losing weight becomes straightforward. Utilize bands in your exercise program, such as in a full-body circuit. This might entail performing a resistance band chest press, followed by band squats, back rows, and chest presses. Long-term weight loss is facilitated by doing this because it simultaneously builds muscle and burns calories.

- **Older Adults**

Standard weights at the gym might be difficult and hard on your body for those who are close to or above the age of 60. Without going overboard, resistance bands help preserve muscle mass and strength. According to research, strengthening exercises utilizing elastic tubes are a practical and efficient way to increase strength in persons over the age of 65. Resistance bands are suggested by Johns Hopkins Medicine as one of the safest ways to strengthen bones and combat osteoporosis.

- **Athletes**

Bands aid athletes in getting ready for motions in all planes, enhancing power and strength while reducing the risk of injuries. Daniel Sanchez, the 2004 National Boxing Champion, noted that "resistance bands are the best thing available for building strength and speed. They are very helpful for my training, particularly with my shadow boxing, punching speed, and even toning without the use of weights. You can take them with you wherever you go and get a good workout no matter where you are. Bands would always be my first choice if I had to choose between dumbbells and weights."

- **Pregnant Women**

For better energy, sleep, mood, and labor preparation during pregnancy, exercise is crucial. However you shouldn't start a rigorous weight-training regimen at this time. High repetitions (15–20) and resistance bands are excellent for light muscular toning. You may easily target your key muscles by alternating between one light and one medium band.

Main Types of Resistance Bands and their Benefits

The five distinct types of bands will be discussed in detail, along with their advantages;

1. **Power resistance bands (aka loop bands)**

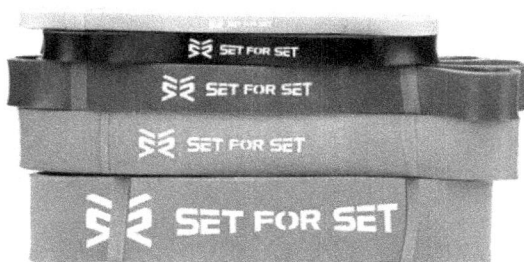

In essence, power resistance loop bands resemble enormous rubber bands. They are a set of continuous flat loops that can be used in numerous ways.

You can use loop bands for full-body exercises (like shoulder presses, thrusters, squats, etc.), bodyweight assistance (like dips, muscle ups, pull-ups, etc.), static stretching (elevated stretch and novel stretching postures you'd otherwise have difficulties with), physical rehabilitation (like those having leg, knee, and back problems), and warm-ups (resistance band bench press, resistance band squats, etc.). You can also fasten resistance bands to a bar or pole for pushing and pulling activities.

In general, you can use power loop bands for all types of exercise, especially bodybuilding and athletic-focused exercises. They provide you with the ability in working through all three planes of motion, making them very versatile. The band's width is what differentiates the sizes. The degree of resistance is determined by breadth.

The bands have widths ranging from 0.25 to 2.5 inches. Therefore, you would have around 5 to 175 lbs of resistance if you had all the different sizes.

The band sizes and resistance levels for the SET FOR SET brands are listed below for reference:

- #1 Yellow (½") – (41" x 0.5" x 0.18") 5 to 30 lbs
- #2 Black (7/8") – (41" x 0.85" x 0.18") 20 to 55 lbs
- #3 Blue (1 ¼") – (41" x 1.25" x 0.18") 35 to 70 lbs
- #4 Green (1 ¾") – (41" x 1.75" x 0.18") 45 to 115 lbs
- #5 Gray (2 ½") – (41" x 2.5" x 0.18") 60 to 170 lbs

Loop Band's Benefits

- Hypertrophy
- Enduring power
- Explosiveness
- Muscle power coordination and balance stability
- Being leaner
- Flexibility
- Rehabilitation for a greater range of motion and mobility
- Limited joint effects

- Unilateral motions and multiplanar exercises

2. Tube Resistance Bands With Handles

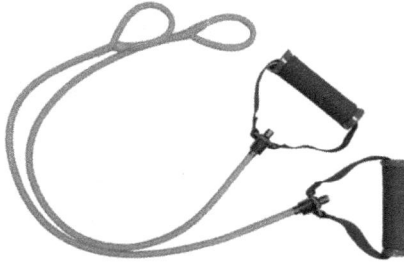

Resistance bands with handles on both ends are designed to resemble activities done with gym equipment like dumbbells. They quickly secure to the door or a pole or bar.

They are beneficial for pressing and pulling activities like shoulder presses, back rows, chest presses, and curls. They are also beneficial for courses like P90X. Tube resistance bands are excellent for people who don't have access to a gym or who like to exercise outside and want something straightforward and conveniently portable because they may work all of your muscle groups.

Sizes/resistance: A set of tube bands typically provides 10 to 50 pounds of resistance. The resistance of the tubes depends on their thickness.

The Advantages Of Tube Resistance Banding

- Skeletal power
- Hypertrophy
- Enduring power
- Improve Motion Spherical
- Losing weight Rehabilitation
- Limited joint effect

3. **Rubber Mini-Bands & Fabric Non-Slip Hip Circle Bands**

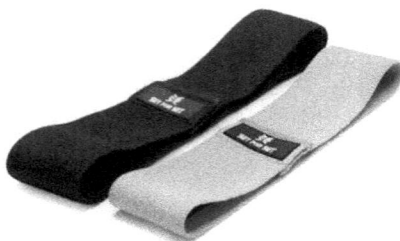

Mini bands are significantly narrower and shorter than loop bands. The mini bands in modern innovations are fabric oriented for improved comfortability and to ensure the band does not roll up, which occurs mostly with the very thin brand of mini bands (the non-slip fabric bands are preferable).

With mini bands, your lower body (and with some workouts, your upper body as well) can be strengthened and stabilized. By placing them around your ankles or just over your knees, you may achieve tremendous hip and glute movement. They are handy for weightlifting as well. You may improve your stability, activate your core, keep a great form, and add more tension and hip activation when you use mini to perform exercises like leg, squats, and hip thrusts extensions.

Like the majority of other bands, mini bands are very effective in strengthening the joints of the shoulder and addressing shoulder problems as well as the elbow.

If you love calisthenics, then mini bands would be a perfect option to get your body ready for activities, such as muscle-ups and handstands. Those who frequent the gym know that mini bands are generally used in a plethora of exercises. This shows how effective and adaptive they are.

Per their size and resistance, mini band sets are commonly categorized as light, medium, heavy, and very heavy. Their resistance is at least five pounds and up to fifty pounds or more. The length and thickness of these bands will vary based on their resistance, but they are all designed to be wrapped around the legs.

Warm-ups are a benefit of mini bands.

4. Light Therapy Resistance Bands

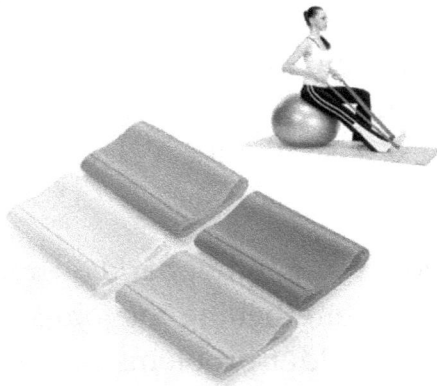

Therapy bands are dubbed "free bands" because they don't loop (however, they can be tied to form a knot or loop); they are thin, light, and quite long, approximately 7 ft. Therapy bands are mostly made for those recovering from an injury and need to build strength and seniors who want a very low-impact exercise. Furthermore, they work well when paired with Pilates and fat-burning workouts. Most women use light therapy bands to tone their muscles in this way.

They can also be utilized for static stretching after a workout activity and for dynamic stretching before a workout activity.

Sizes/Resistance: A set of therapy bands will typically provide 3–10 pounds of resistance.

Light Therapy Resistance Band's Benefits:

- Physical therapy and recovery
- Losing weight
- Toned muscles
- Strengthening of muscles (for beginners or people with muscle weakness)
- Flexibility

5. **Figure 8 Bands**

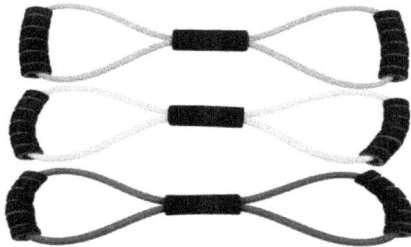

Figure 8 bands have the precise shape that the name implies. On either side of the figure-8 design, there are soft handles. To target your upper and lower body, they stretch as far as you'd need them to. Figure 8 bands can be used for lateral motions similarly to mini bands and similarly to tube resistance bands to imitate exercises with machines and dumbbells. They work well for pushing and pulling exercises in the sagittal and lateral planes of motion.

Sizes/Resistance: A set of figure 8 bands will typically provide 8–20 pounds of resistance.

Figure-8 band advantages:

- Physical therapy and recovery
- Losing weight
- Toned muscles
- Strengthening of muscles
- Enduring power
- Stability with one-sided motions

Tips When Buying Resistance Bands

There are a few additional attributes you can look for in a resistance band besides type and color. You may choose the ideal resistance band for your workout and yourself with the aid of the attributes discussed below.

- **Length:** Resistance bands come in a range of lengths. Some of them are tiny and can't even extend past arm's length. Others are fairly comprehensive. Lean toward lengthier options if you're not sure which length to choose. Longer bands are typically easier to knot, wrap, or even cut if necessary, as opposed to short bands, which are more difficult to alter in any way.
- **Material:** Although most resistance bands are comprised of rubber-like tubing, the exact materials utilized can vary substantially. A resistance band has a higher chance of tearing or stretching out of shape depending on the material. Generally speaking, it is wise to stick with true rubber latex blends of bands.
- **Handles:** You should make a decision regarding your preference for the type of handles you want (if you want handles at all). However, you will undoubtedly need handles if you frequently perform activities that are similar to dumbbells. Following that, you should choose how soft and

grip-able those handles should be. If you've never worked with resistance bands before, choose softer handles to avoid developing calluses.

Resistance Band Colors and Levels

To show what level of resistance they produce, resistance bands come in a variety of colors. Resistance bands can vary greatly in weight. Whatever the brand, most resistance bands generally follow the color scheme below. But other companies might have their own color scheme, particularly for more odd bands like therapy bands and loop bands.

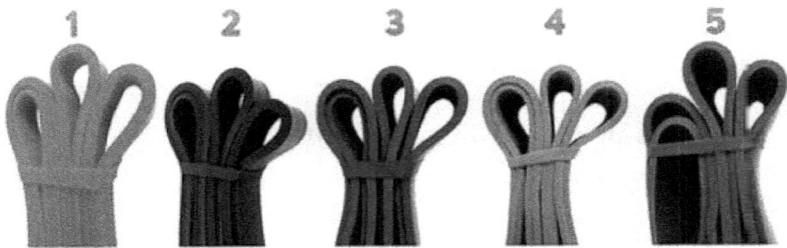

1. The Red Resistance Band

This color band is the thinnest and the most stretchable resistance band. Although all practitioners continue to utilize it, it is ideal for individuals just beginning resistance band training because the band's small weight enables it to target muscle regions that don't require a lot of resistance to remain active. To exercise your shoulder or shin muscles, for instance, you may use a red band.

Level of Resistance: Light-duty resistance

Muscles to target: Shoulders and shins

2. The Black Resistance Band

Red resistance bands are slightly more elastic than black ones, but overall, black bands offer a higher level of tension. They are categorized as "medium resistance" due to this, making them a decent middle-of-the-road option. To target particular muscle areas that perform well with medium resistance, such as your triceps or biceps, you could utilize your black band if you feel that you have graduated from your red band.

Level of Resistance: Medium-duty resistance

Muscles to target: Triceps and biceps

3. The Purple Resistance Band

The next level up from red is the medium-to-heavy purple resistance band. It should only be utilized by people who have a lot of muscle tone or want to concentrate on broad, muscular groups rather than individual muscles. For instance, you may exercise your legs with a purple resistance band.

Level of Resistance: Medium-duty to heavy-duty resistance

Muscles to target: Legs, chest, and back

4. The Green Resistance Band

Strong and unyielding are the green resistance bands. Similar to the purple resistance bands, they should only be used on major muscle areas or following practice with stretchier bands.

Level of Resistance: Heavyduty resistance

Muscles to target: Back, chest, and legs

5. The Blue Resistance Band

The hardest resistance bands to use are the blue ones. They are incredibly stiff and difficult to stretch. Before working with these bands, ensure you have developed your strength. Blue resistance bands are a terrific option for partnered or paired exercises since they are so challenging to stretch out, requiring both you and the other party to pull against the band.

Level of Resistance: Heavy-duty resistance

Muscles to target: Legs

Chapter 2

Getting Started With Resistance Bands Exercises

Workout Gears

For a resistance band workout, not much in terms of gear and clothing is required. Below are some of what you'll need:

Resistance Band

This one should be apparent, right? Having several resistance bands with varying levels of resistance (or stretchiness) is ideal. There are many available designs, which have been covered previously in chapter 1. Pick the option that is most convenient and pleasant to use. (You can make this decision by evaluating the workouts you would perform with the bands)

Clothing You Can Conveniently Sweat and Move In

Dress in breathable, loose-fitting clothing that won't restrict your movement and won't feel burdensome as your body warms up.

The following gears and equipment can be used as part of your workout session, but they surely make some exercises easier to complete.

- **Sneakers:**

Many resistance band workouts can be performed without shoes. However, think about lacing up if you're in a place where you risk slipping or if wearing shoes makes you feel more confident, stable, and grounded.

- **Yoga Mat:**

If you are performing workouts on the ground and you are on a hard surface, adding some padding, like a yoga mat, can help avoid tripping.

- **Towel:**

This is an obvious need when working out. So, ensure you add this to your list of gears.

Safety Precautions and Tips

Resistance bands are often less risky compared to weights; however, caution must be applied in general when exercising. You are considerably less likely to get injured and can achieve your fitness objectives quicker when you're cautious with your bands. Let's look at some important safety precautions you should be mindful of when exercising with your resistance bands.

- **Maintain Proper Bodily Alignment**

Even though it gives your body more strength, you shouldn't ever be slouched over in an unsupportable position while performing resistance exercises. Instead, keep your posture at a steady level. While working out, your knees should be bent slightly rather than locked. Allow your spine to maintain its natural bend while keeping your shoulders and hips in alignment.

- **Try Working Out Without a Band**

If you're undertaking an exercise that you've not done before, first get some practice without using the band. By doing so, you can learn the correct movement without taxing your muscles. Start increasing the resistance until you are confident and at ease with the workout.

- **Remember to breathe!**

There is frequently a desire to keep your breath while you contract your muscles during any type of resistance or strength exercise. Defy this temptation and take deep, even breaths. Exhale instead of inhaling or keeping your breath when the resistance levels increase.

- **Avoid Locking Your Joints**

You're likely exerting so much resistance if you notice that your joints lock up when the band increases. Regardless of whether the resistance band is totally stretched, your joints must always be somewhat bent. Otherwise, you'll risk straining your muscles excessively and having them injured in the process.

- **Don't Be In a Rush**

Don't move on to harder bands too fast. Rather, spend time to make certain that you fully understand a band color before deciding to go on to the next level. As a general rule, you should perform an exercise for 3 sets of 10 to 15 reps before attempting it with another band.

- **An Extended or Tensed Resistance Band Must Be Released with Caution**

A resistance band that has previously been extended will return to its original position (toward you) when you release it. When this happens, the band handle could hit you in the face, which is not a pleasant experience. Never let go of your band before the tension has been released.

- **Do Not Overuse and Overextend the Band**

Resistance bands that are continuously layered run the risk of breaking after several years when used often. However, unlike the "pop" that occurs when single-layered bands rupture, the break for a multi-layer band is usually slow. A little tear is where a multi-layer band would first show signs before it breaks. Therefore, if your bands are old, ensure to examine them before utilizing them. Avoid bands with a single layer as well.

Also, if you stretch a resistance band beyond its recommended use or utilize it on a rough surface, it may break. Continuous multilayering bands may often be stretched up to 2.5 to 3 times their length with no problems. For anchors like wooden beams, a towel should be placed around them first before wrapping the band around the towel to protect them from the effect of rough surfaces.

Overall, you shouldn't be scared of them breaking for a very long time if they are used properly (and not used on rough surfaces). Before a break occurs, you'll be fully aware that a new band is required.

33

- **Examine Your Band Before You Use it**

Check your band carefully every time before you start your workout. Examine it for any rips or frays that could cause more serious harm while working out. You wouldn't want your band to suddenly snap as tension is applied to it.

Avoid Keeping Your Band in Sunny or Muggy Places

As soon as you finish using your band, wipe the handles. Additionally, avoid keeping it in places where the rubber is likely to swell or support bacterial growth. If stored in a cool, dry area, your band will last for a while.

Warming Up

We are all aware of how critical a rigorous warm-up is to reducing injury risk and improving performance. Resistance bands are excellent gears to use in the warm-up procedure. Warm-ups are designed to elevate your heart rate and prime your distinct muscle groups for the workout activities that will follow thereafter.

The full-body resistance band use-ups below use the resistance bands' regulated resistance to get you ready for a workout activity. For a full-body workout that builds muscle, you could also do the entire warm-ups about 3 to 4 times or break it into several supersets.

Front Raise x10 Reps

- Wrap the band underneath your two feet.
- Position yourself vertically as you hold the opposite end of the band.
- Lift the band upward until your hands are at the height of your shoulder while maintaining a straight back, straight arms, and tucked-in shoulders.
- After a 1 sec brief pause, restart the activity.

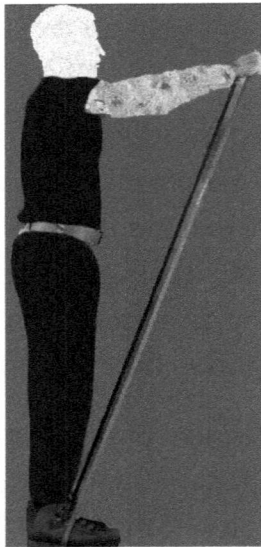

Side Raise x10 Reps

- Stand straight while holding the band with one foot.
- Take hold of the band's other end.
- Lift the band to the height of your shoulder while maintaining a chest up and bent elbow position, lowering it back to the starting position.

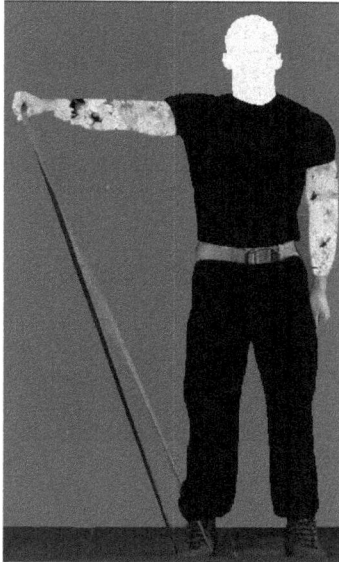

Bent-Over Row x10 Reps

- Use both of your feet to stand on one edge of the resistance band.

- Grab the band firmly while hip-hinging.
- Squeeze the blades of your shoulder, pushing your elbows back to your sides.
- Take a little pause for a second, then straighten your arms to begin afresh.

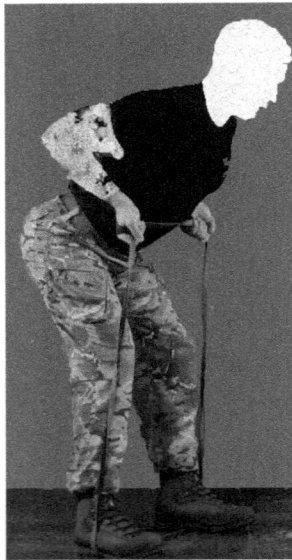

Overhead Squats x10 Reps

- Grab the band with a shoulder-width grip.
- Hold firmly, putting the band against your hand's heels.
- Your elbows should remain just beneath your hands for the entire workout.

- Pull the band over your head, locking your elbows.
- Hold your arms in the overhead position as you squat down.
- Go as low as you possibly can while maintaining a flawless form, then rise to your feet.

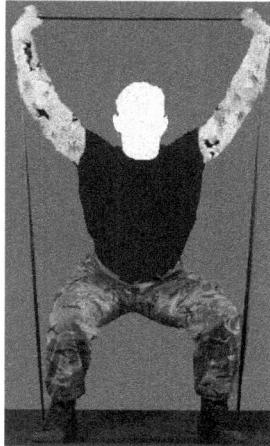

Triceps Kickbacks x10 Reps

- Grab the band around your back and secure one end of it to the floor with your heel.
- Raise your elbows such that your upper arms are aligned with the floor.

- Stretch your arms completely with the band's opposite end right around your back, and revert to the starting point.

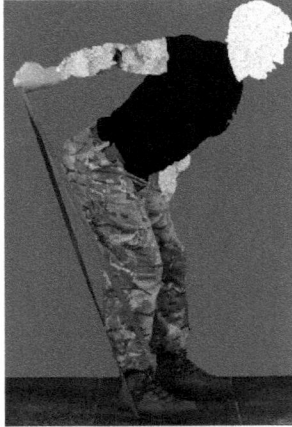

Workout Routine

Beginners can undertake resistance band exercises for about 3 to 4x per week.

If you opt for a 4-day split, then your schedule can be as follows:

1. First Day: Chest/Abs
2. Second Day: Glutes/Legs
3. Third Day: Rest
4. Fourth Day: Shoulders/Arms

5. Fifth Day: Back/Abs
6. Sixth Day: Rest
7. Seventh Day: Rest

Or you can do the upper/lower body split as given below:

1. First Day: Upper Body
2. Second Day: Lower Body
3. Third Day: Rest
4. Fourth Day: Upper Body
5. Fifth Day: Lower Body
6. Sixth Day: Rest
7. Seventh Day: Rest

However, if you opt for a full body exercise routine, then resistance band exercises are ideal to be undertaken every other day.

Intermediate and experienced athletes can exercise up to 6x per week. If you have a high degree of fitness, you probably don't expect me to explain how to create a workout routine. The resistance band exercises discussed subsequently should provide you with all the motivation you require to get started.

Whether you are a beginner, intermediate or advanced athlete, ensure you always pay attention to your body. While attempting to maintain the highest possible workout frequency, you should also avoid overtraining. Do a brief high-intensity interval training (HIIT) or cardio workout on your rest day if you feel particularly energetic.

Workout Programming Sets and Reps

Below are the resistance band workout programming sets and reps to adhere to when performing the resistance band exercises (per muscle group) to be discussed in the subsequent chapters. I have taken the time to divide the exercises in subsequent chapters into different muscle groups, and I also included an illustration of an excellent full-body fat-burning exercise. Workouts that target specific muscle groups sound more logical if you're trying to develop your muscles. Still, full-body exercises like those discussed in the next chapter are the best option since they burn the most calories and can help you tone up and get in better shape.

That said, every set or round in a circuit workout program, for instance, using resistance band exercises, would be rigorous. If you want to gain muscle and lose fat, try to get the most out of your time under tension. You can also engage in a challenging workout plan. It may consist of 4 sets x 20 reps for some people and 3 sets x 10 reps for others. Be mindful of your body and push yourself as much as possible. If you intend building your muscle, make an effort to increase the difficulty of your workouts every week. You can gradually overload with bands; you just need to think more creatively than you'd with free weights, i.e., not just adding extra weight or resistance.

Without further ado, let's look at the workout programming reps and sets you should adhere to for each muscle group exercise discussed in the following chapters.

Resistance Band Chest/Abs Workout

- Chest Press – 4 sets of 10 to 15 reps
- Banded Push-ups – 4 sets of 10 to 20 reps
- Chest Fly – 4 sets of 10 to 15 reps
- Plank Liftoffs – 3 sets of 10 reps (lifting all the limbs in the sequence constitute 1 rep)
- Crossbody Chop – 3 sets of 10 reps (on both sides)
- Hallow Hold – 3 sets of 30 to 60 secs

Resistance Band Legs/Glutes/Calves Workout

- Power Squats – 4 sets of 10 to 12 reps
- Sumo Squats – 4 sets of 10 to 12 reps
- Good Mornings – 4 sets of 10 reps
- Split Squats – 3 sets of 10 reps on both sides
- Hip Bridge – 3 sets of 10 to 12 reps
- Lateral Walks – 3 sets of 10 reps both way

Resistance Band Shoulders/Arms Workout

- Reverse Curl | Press – 4 sets of 10 to 12 reps
- Kneeling Overhead Press – 4 sets of 10 to 15 reps
- Lateral Raise – 3 sets of 10 reps
- Upright Rows – 3 sets of 10 reps
- Bicep Curls – 3 sets of 10 to 15 reps
- Triceps Extensions – 3 sets of 10 to 15 reps

Resistance Band Back/Abs Workout

- Pull Aparts – 4 sets of 15 reps
- Single Arm Bent Over Row – 4 sets of 10 to 15 reps
- Pulldown | Shrug – 4 sets of 10 to 15 reps
- Hinge | Row | Squat – 3 sets of 10 reps

Full Body Resistance Band Workout

- Thrusters – Complete as many hinge, row, and squat exercises in five minutes, and only take breaks when necessary.
- Hinge | Row | Squat – Complete as many hinge, row, and squat exercises in five minutes, and only take breaks when necessary.
- Circuit – Perform each of the exercises below one after another, resting only after all the three exercises have been completed for the given time (rest for thirty secs, repeating a total of three rounds)

  - Reverse Curl | Press – Perform for 30 secs
  - Power Squats – Perform for 30 secs
  - Banded Push Ups – Perform for 30 secs (dropping to your knees if necessary)

Gradual Overload with Bands

If you seek to gain muscle and strength, you must increase the intensity of your workouts every week or two weeks. For this to happen, the number of reps can be increased, extra sets should be added, extra exercise should be added, rest time should be decreased, or simply use the next resistance band level from the one currently used (this is the final step).

Simply put, increase the level of difficulty with each workout. Track your workouts so you can challenge yourself a bit more the next time.

Slowly, but surely. Consistency is key.

If all you want to do is stay fit, stay in shape, and have fun, then test different workout routines, try something new, and don't bother too much about adhering to a rigid gradual overload regimen.

In general, the workouts discussed in the subsequent chapters are excellent for increasing muscular strength, endurance, and weight loss. If you wish to gain muscle, you should increase your time spent under tension and eat a great deal of protein. If losing weight is your objective, cutting back on carbs and keeping your rest time shorter will help you achieve this.

Chapter 3

Full Body

Thrusters

Complete as many hinge, row, and squat exercises in five minutes, and only take breaks when necessary

Steps

1. Place your foot on the bands, ensuring it's around your shoulder width.
2. Holding the band shoulder-width apart, your palms should face out, starting at the level of your collar bone.

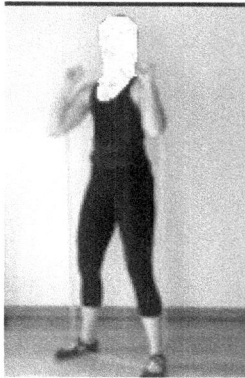

3. Squat down.

4. As you stand up from the squat, press yourself up and raise the band overhead.

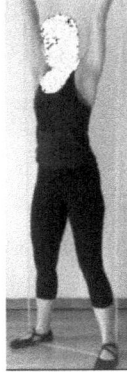

Target Muscles: Quads, glutes, core, shoulders, triceps, and hamstrings

Hinge – Row – Squat

Complete as many hinge, row, and squat exercises in five minutes, and only take breaks when necessary.

Steps

1. Stand on the band and hold the ends with your palms pointing inwards toward one another

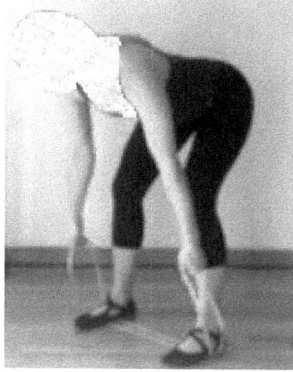

2. Adjust into the hinge position, such as a stiff-legged, deadlift starting point.

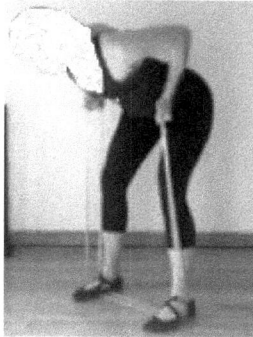

3. Perform a row (completely contract your muscles), then gradually lower the bands.

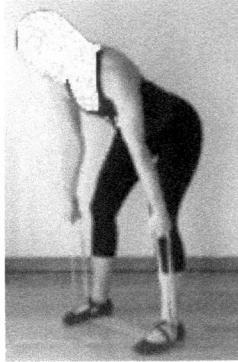

4. Raise your body to a balanced spine standing position as you'd a stiff-legged deadlift.

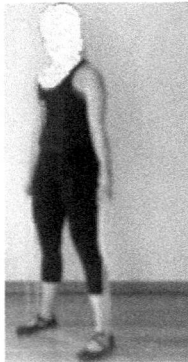

5. Squat down.

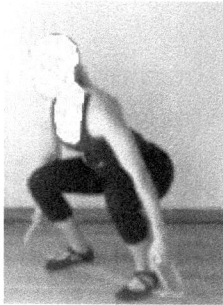

6. After squatting, stand up.
7. Hinge and go again

Target Muscles: Quads, Glutes, Back, Core, Hamstrings, and Biceps

Lateral Lunge Upright Row

Steps

1. Start by positioning both of your feet on each side at about a foot wider than the width of your shoulder.
2. With your right foot, step on the band while holding it in your left hand with your palm downward.

3. Pull the band until it is taut and your left hand is aligned in the direction of your left shoulder.

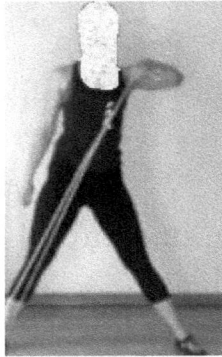

4. Lateral lunge to the side on your right, bringing your left hand downward in the direction of your right foot.

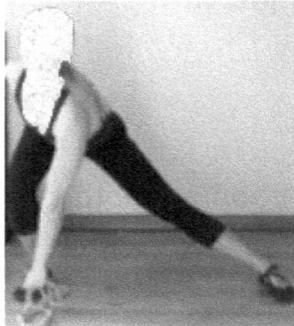

5. Bring the band back up to your shoulder level as you stand. Keep your elbow raised to align with your shoulder's tops.

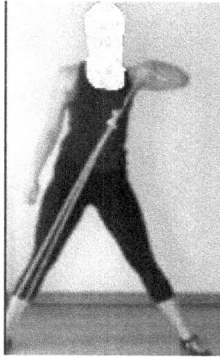

6. Keep at it for 3 sets of 10 reps each.
7. Then repeat on the other side.

Target Muscles: Hamstrings, Glutes, Quads, Shoulders, Back/Rear Delts, Core/Oblique Slings, and Outer Hips

Chapter 4

Legs

Power Squats

Steps

1. Place your feet on the band and ensure its width and that of your shoulders are apart or with your feet a little wider; hold the ends of the band while your palms face inwards toward one another.

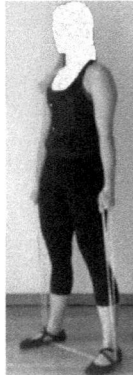

2. Squat down, exploding back up.
3. Repeat for 4 sets of 10 to 12 reps each

Target Muscles: Quads and Glutes

Split Squats

Steps

1. Place your right foot on the band, wrapping the band around your head just along your traps and upper back
2. Reposition your left foot such that it is backward and straight, and your feet are flat on the ground with your heels up.

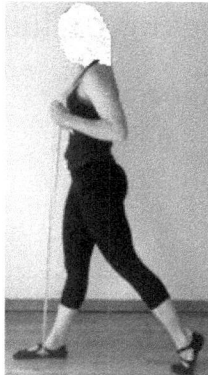

3. Squat down such that your knee is just above the ground's surface (about 1-inch).

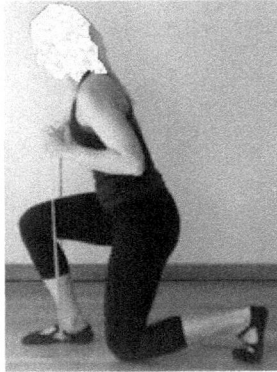

4. Squat back up. Your body ought to be moving up and down in a linear fashion.
5. Continue for 3 sets of 10 reps each
6. Replicate on the other side.

Target Muscles: Hamstrings, Glutes, and Quads

Sumo Squats

Steps

1. Put the resistance band over your feet and squat down into a sumo posture (i.e., your feet

around 3 to 4 ft away from each other with your toes pointing out at 45-degrees).

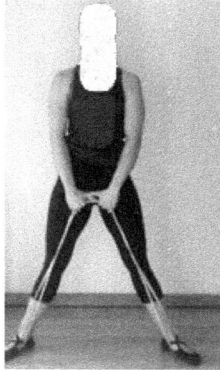

2. Squat down with your hands at your midline; try to maintain a neutral spine.

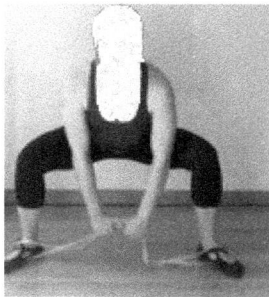

3. When your glutes and knees are somewhat parallel to each other, squat back up and tighten your glutes at the top
4. Repeat for 4 sets of 10 to 12 reps each

Target Muscles: Glutes, Hamstrings, and Quads

Chapter 5

Glutes

Good Mornings

Steps

1. Your feet should be hip-width apart when you step on the band.
2. Place the band over your lower traps after pulling it around your head.

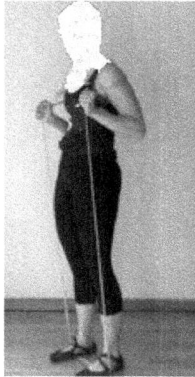

3. Utilizing your hip hinge, relax your body until your back, and the ground are parallel to each other while keeping your knees slightly bent. Your back should not bend; it should be straight.

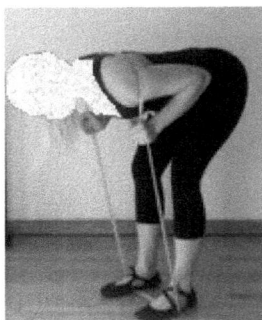

4. Your back should be lifted back up into an upright posture, then squeeze your glutes, keeping your spine balanced and your legs upright.
5. Ensure to maintain a straight band always to keep the tension. To achieve this, pull up with your hands on the band.
6. Repeat for 4 sets of 10 reps each

Target Muscles: Erector Spinae (lower back), Glutes, and Hamstrings

Lateral Walk

Steps

1. Put both of your feet on the band while keeping them about hip- to shoulder-width apart.
2. Take hold of the band with your hands at around the hip level after crossing it, forming an "X." Ensure that the band is tight.

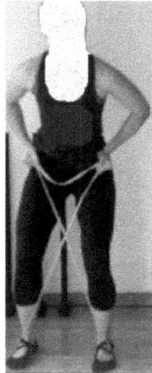

3. Take a foot-long step to the right with your right foot as you hold everything taut. Then, bring your left foot to the right, putting your feet back to shoulder-width distance.

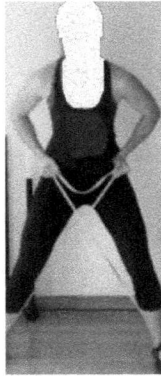

4. Repeat these steps; right foot, left foot, for 3 sets of 10 reps each, and then repeat the same on the other side.

Note: As you perform the side steps, assume a half-squat posture to make it more challenging. Additionally, it enhances knee and hip stability, which is excellent for preventing injuries.

Target Muscles: Thighs, Glutes, and Hips (adductors).

Hip Bridge

Steps

1. Lay down on the ground facing up with your bent knees and flat feet on the ground. Your front knee and back heels should be in alignment.

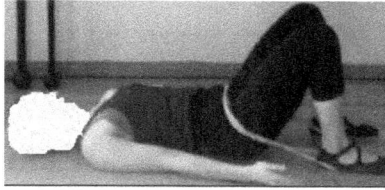

2. Stamp your heels on the loop ends of the band as you place them in front of your pelvic bone as soon as the band is secured. Raise your hips till your torso is in alignment with your legs.

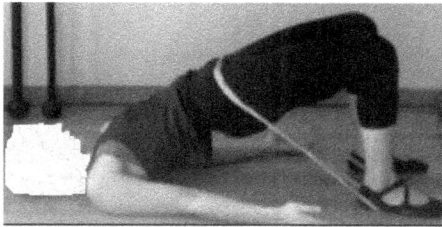

3. Repeat for 3 sets of 10 to 12 reps each, gently lowering down gradually to achieve eccentric contraction.

Target Muscles: Hip flexors/Psoas, Glutes, Hamstrings, Core/ Lower Back

A Request from the Author:

Hey, I trust you'are having a fascinating read. Please do share your feedback with me!

I'd be forever thankful if you could spend only 60 seconds writing a brief product review of this book on Amazon.

\>> To post a brief review, click here.

Thanks so much.

Chapter 6

Shoulders

Upright Row

Steps

1. Stand on the band with your shoulder and feet distant apart.
2. The band should be crossed to form an "X," grabbing it with your hands at around the hip level. Ensure that the band is tight.

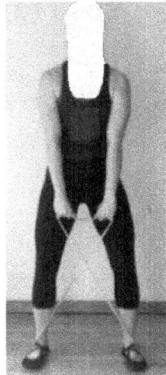

3. Lift your hands such that your elbows and shoulders are aligned and parallel to the ground. The level of your hands should be lifted to be around your shoulder height.

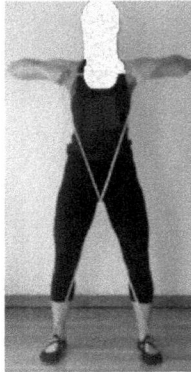

4. Bring the band slowly back down and repeat for 3 sets of 10 reps each.

Target Muscles: Deltoid and Traps

Kneeling Overhead Press

Steps

1. Kneel on the ground or a yoga mat with the band underneath your knees.

2. Hold the bands with your palms facing out and raise them to your upper chest.

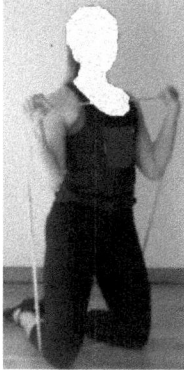

3. Press up overhead.

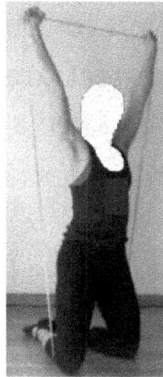

4. Gradually bring the band back to chest level and repeat for 4 sets of 10 to 15 reps each.

Target Muscles: Core, Triceps, Deltoids, and a bit of Upper Chest

Lateral Raise

Steps

1. Stand on the band using your right foot, grabbing it along with your palms faced against one another and your hands slightly broader than your shoulder width.
2. Reposition your left foot backward such that it is upright and your feet are flat on the floor with your heels up; each knee a little bent.

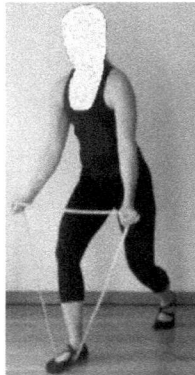

3. Lift your arms and hands so they are roughly at face level with the band. Be sure to keep your elbows raised but below your shoulders. Keep your shoulders back and your chest up as well.

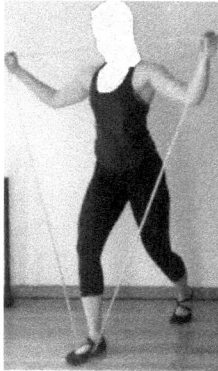

4. Return slowly to the beginning point, and then, as the band is about to slack, bring it back up and ensure to maintain the tension throughout.
5. Repeat for 3 sets of 10 reps each.

Target Muscles: Middle Deltoids (as well as your front and back delts), and Upper Traps, Serratus Anterior, and Rotator Cuff Complex.

Chapter 7

Chest

Chest Press

Steps

1. Take a split position with both feet planted firmly on the floor

2. Put the band over your head and beneath your arms (or over your arms, making it very challenging).

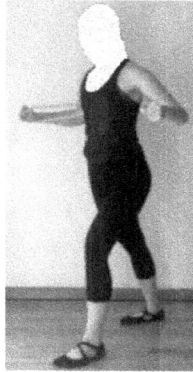

3. Using your hands to hold the ends of the bands, press forward and a little upward with your palms downward. Your hands, arms, and shoulder should form a vertical line.

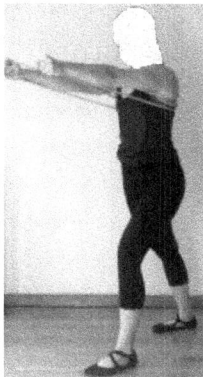

4. Slowly make your way back to where you started, then do it again for 4 sets of 10 to 15 reps each; slower is preferable because the eccentric contraction will be more productive at activating the muscles.

Target Muscles: Shoulders, Triceps, and Chest

Chest Fly

Steps

1. Assume a split position, bringing one foot forward and the other backward with both feet grounded firmly.
2. The band should be wrapped over your back and beneath your arms (or over your arms, making it very challenging)

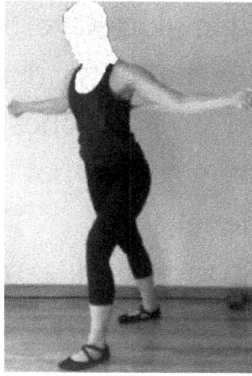

3. Using your hands to hold the ends of the bands with your palms opposite one another, pull your hands to your front and middle such that your hands extend forward. Elbows should be bent very slightly. Align your hands with your sternum such that it's a little beneath the level of your shoulder.

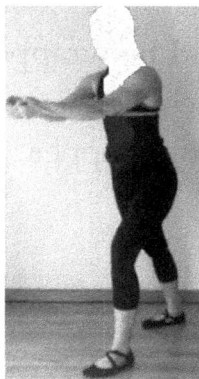

4. Once the band makes a vertical line across your chest with your hands and arms at your sides, gradually open up your chest (sense the stretch); still, your elbows somewhat bent and the band at a lower chest level.
5. Return your hands and arms to the front and middle of your body (the starting point) using the same movement above, then repeat for 4 sets of 10 to 15 reps each.

Target Muscles: Triceps, Shoulders, and Chest

Banded Push-up

Steps

1. The band should be wrapped over your back. To make it very challenging, wrap the resistance band across your upper arms or below your arms.

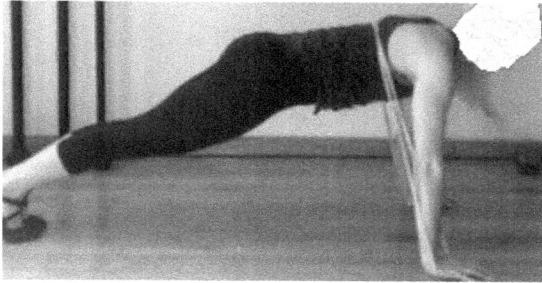

2. Position yourself in the push-up posture and execute a conventional push-up. To engage your muscles efficiently, try exploding up and moving down gradually.

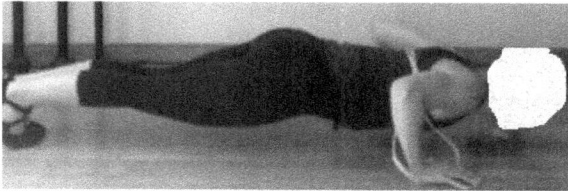

3. Repeat for 4 sets of 10 to 20 reps each

Target Muscles: Abs, Triceps, Shoulders, and Chest

Chapter 8

Back

Pull Aparts

Steps

1. Raise your arms to align with the height of your shoulder and hold onto the band fist tight with your hands and shoulder distance apart. The tension should be constant in an ideal situation, even from the start.

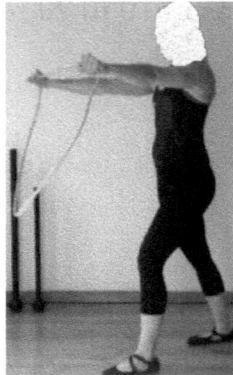

2. Push the band apart, bringing your arms to your sides. Feel the muscles in your shoulder blades contracting and squeezing collectively; pay keen attention to the activation of your posterior delts muscle.

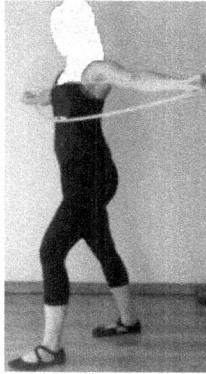

3. Return gradually to your starting point.
4. Repeat for 4 sets of 15 reps each.

Target Muscles: Rhomboids, middle traps, and posterior deltoids

Pulldown – Shrug

Steps

1. Kneel down

2. Hold the band with your hands spaced roughly three feet away, bringing your arms right over your head to create a "Y."

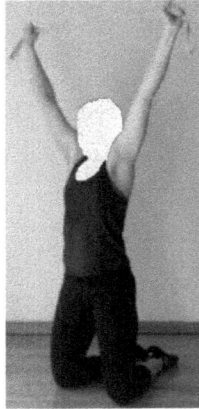

3. Shrug up, pulling your arms down.

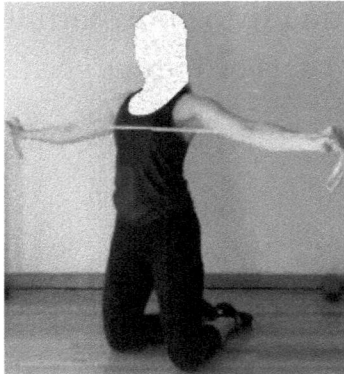

4. Gradually lift your arms again to create the Y position, shrug, and repeat 4 sets of 10 to 15 reps.

The band will move in a straight, upward, and downward vertical direction.

Target Muscles: Biceps, Traps, and Latissimus Dorsi (lats)

Single Arm Bent Over Row

Steps

1. Position yourself by standing in a split posture with your front foot on the band and your back foot on your foot's ball, bending your knees likewise.
2. Wrap the band over your hand on the exact side your front foot is positioned. Your back shouldn't be curved but straight.

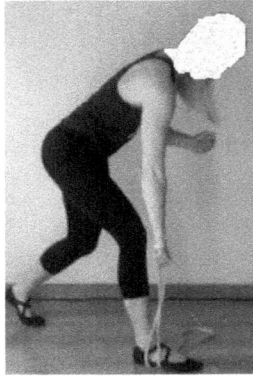

3. Pull the band upward and slightly backward such that your elbow extends past your back and your arm, almost forming a 90-degree angle. Your whole body should be kept tight on this.

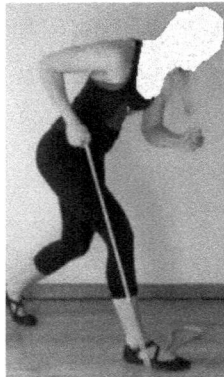

4. Lower the band back down gradually, repeating for 4 sets of 10 to 15 reps each.

Target Muscles: Teres Major & Minor, Lats, Biceps, Core, Infraspinatus, Traps, and Posterior Delts

Chapter 9

Arms

Biceps Curl

Steps

1. Hold onto the band a little broader than the width of your shoulder as you step on the band with your feet and shoulder distance apart. A square shape will be made by the band from the ground to your upper thigh

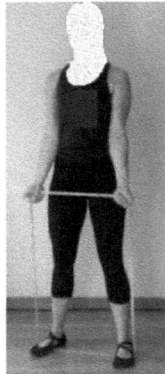

2. Curl up the band in straight form while keeping your arms upright. Maintain an outward-facing palm a little bit to add more tension to your biceps. Nonetheless, a bicep curl with your hands can likewise be achieved when your hand is in an overhand or neutral posture.

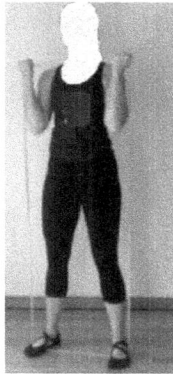

3. Lower down gradually, repeating for 3 sets of 10 to 15 reps each.

Target Muscles: Forearms and Biceps

Kneeling Triceps Extension

Steps

1. Kneel down with the bands beneath your knees.
2. Hold onto the band's top end with both hands placed on top of one another.
   Your elbows should be pointed directly upward in line with your shoulders, and your hands resting right below the base of your neck.

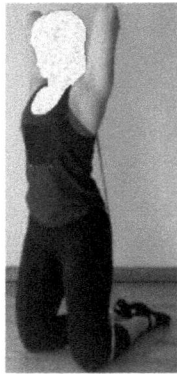

3. Make an extension by moving your hands up past your head. Just your forearms would move; your elbow and upper arm won't. Concentrate on the triceps.

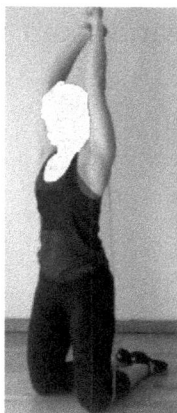

4. Squeeze at the peak when your arms are extended.
5. Gradually move back down, repeating for 3 sets of 10 to 15 reps each.

Target Muscles: Triceps

Reverse Curl – Press

Steps

1. Step on the band with your feet and shoulder distance apart, grabbing onto the band a little wider than the width of your shoulder with your palms towards your body. A square shape will be

formed by the band from the ground up to your upper thigh.

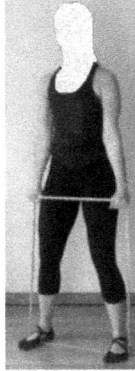

2. Reverse curl the band up to your shoulder level; your palms wouldn't be facing outward.

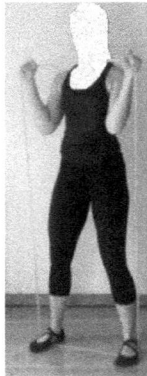

3. Press right over your head.

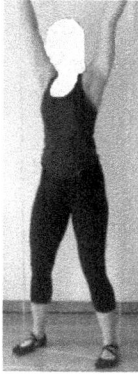

4. Bring the band back to the starting point in a two-step fashion.
5. Repeat for 4 sets of 10 to 12 reps each.

Target Muscles: Shoulders, Biceps, Triceps, and Forearms

The End... Almost!

Hey! This book has come to its last chapter, and I trust you've had a good read thus far.

As a self-published author with a limited advertising budget, I depend on you, my readers, to post a quick review of my book on Amazon because readers hardly post reviews.

So, if you truly liked this book, would you kindly...

Submit a quick review on Amazon by clicking >> here.

Thanks so much.

Chapter 10

Core

Crossbody Chop

Steps

1. Put your right foot over the band with your feet wider than the width of your, then hold onto the band's other end with your hands stacked and pointing inward.
2. Turn to your right side, bending your knees with your left leg bent significantly and in the same direction as your upper body on the right. Your right knee will be below your hands.

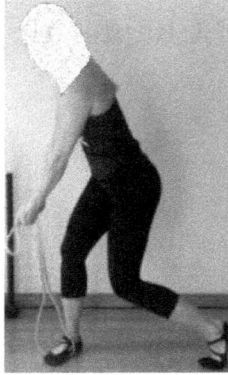

3. Bring the band up, so your body and hips are pointing up to the left while diagonally rotating your body and hips. Straighten your arms and raise them above your head.

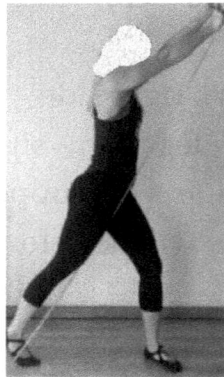

4. Revert gradually in the same direction of movement, continuing for 3 sets of 10 reps each.
5. Repeat on the other side.

Target Muscles: Glutes and Core/Oblique Slings

Hollow Hold

Steps

1. While lying flat on your back, pull your belly button toward the ground by contracting your abdominal muscles.
2. Put the band beneath your feet, then take hold of the other end with both hands. Hold out your arms and legs straight from your body, hands and toes pointed. Maintain a uniform tension on the band.
3. Lift your shoulders and legs gradually off the ground.

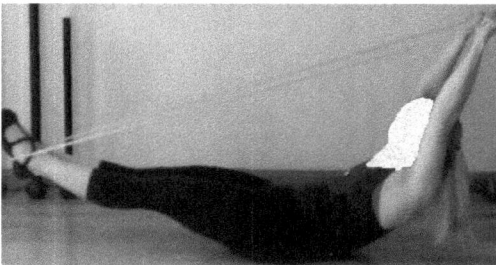

4. Maintain this posture for 3 sets of 30 to 6C secs each.

Resisted Plank Lift-Offs

Steps

1. Put the band over your right foot and loop it over your left hand while positioning yourself in a regular plank posture.

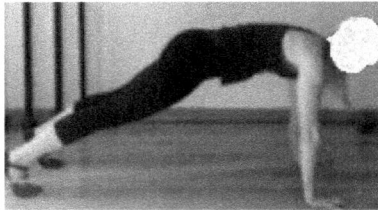

2. Raise your left hand off the ground, holding for 1 or 2 second before lowering it back down.

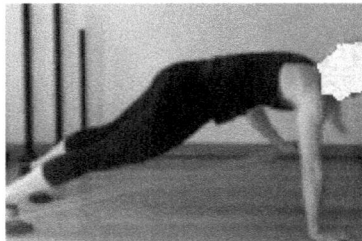

3. Raise your right hand off the ground, holding for 1 or 2 second before lowering it back down.

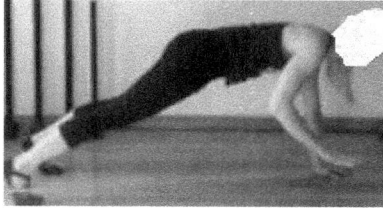

4. Raise your right leg off the ground, holding for 1 or 2 second before lowering it back down.

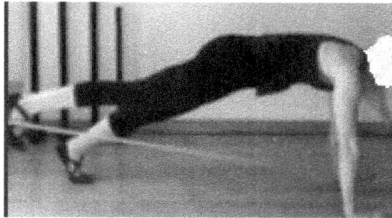

5. Raise your left leg off the ground, holding for 1 or 2 second before lowering it back down.

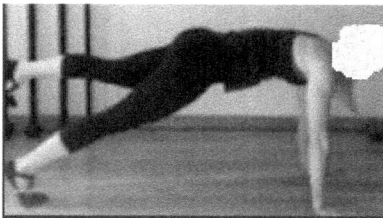

6. Repeat this process for 3 sets of 10 reps each (lifting all the limbs in the sequence constitute 1 rep)

Target Muscles: Hips, Erector Spinae, Quadratus Lumborum, Glutes, Internal and External Obliques, Transverse Abdominis, and Abdominis

Conclusion

Resistance band exercises are a great way to include stretching and strength exercises in your routine for improved body fitness, which every fitness fanatic should engage in at least three times each week, regardless of your present fitness level. Resistance bands are inexpensive and convenient to keep, making them a great piece of equipment worth purchasing. As earlier highlighted, resistance bands are great for more than just at-home workouts. They are also convenient for on-the-go workouts, which is why they can be easily slipped into a bag and brought along with you for a fast workout in a park nearby or when traveling. The resistance band exercises discussed in the pages of this book will not only help you tone your muscles (for those looking to build their muscles) but will also help in burning body fat (for those looking to lose weight) and improving your general body fitness.

What more can I say? All you need to get started with resistance band exercises have been discussed in each chapter, and the exercises have been grouped into distinct muscle groups, making it easy for you to focus on a particular group to work on or on all groups (depending on your fitness objective).

So, I encourage you to take the bull by the horn, get your resistance band if you haven't, and get into that extra fitness mode with the exercises in this book as you work toward achieving your fitness goal.

I wish you all the best!

www.ingramcontent.com/pod-product-compliance
Lightning Source LLC
Chambersburg PA
CBHW071037050426
42335CB00051B/2323